"When you are caring for the well-being of others 80 hours a week, it is easy to forget to care for your own well-being. In <u>50 Simple Things to Save Your Life During Residency</u>, Dr Ben Brown reminds us to care for ourselves and offers practical, attainable and effective ways to do this. Small enough to fit in your pocket, it's like carrying your own doctor in your white coat!"

– Rachel Naomi Remen, M.D. Author of
Kitchen Table Wisdom & My Grandfather's Blessings

"This book saved my night more than once. It was as important for my medical education as any other medical handbook. The entertaining and often profound tips and techniques in this book are a guide for anyone who has struggled to keep a sense of wholeness, joy and love of the healing profession during medical school or residency. I still share the practices and wisdom in Dr. Ben Brown's book with patients and colleagues."

– Heidi Reetz, M.D.

"I have read this handbook many times over. It is filled with invaluable pearls of wisdom gained from years of experience. The book continues to occupy a prominent place on my bookshelf even after residency!"

– Anthony Lim, M.D.

50 SIMPLE THINGS
TO SAVE YOUR LIFE
DURING RESIDENCY
(AND BEYOND)

Ben Brown, M.D.

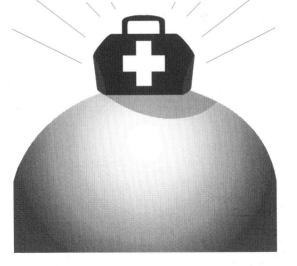

"Peace comes not from the absence of conflict, but from the ability to cope with it." -Anonymous

This book is dedicated to everyone going through this initiation called Residency. May it help you to save your life and keep your dream intact so that when you finish you can go out and do what you are here to do.

You can and will survive ... REALLY!!!

- Dr. Ben

Copyright © IM Publishing
First edition 1995
Second edition 2014
Ben Brown MD

ISBN: 978-1-941587-00-3

Thanks, Ben

Acknowledgments

Thanks to the many people who have helped keep me and my dreams alive.

In particular, I want to thank my Residency classmates, the many residents that have come before and behind and stayed alive, the faculty that still cares, and the friends, teachers, and family that have supported me along the way. Thanks to John and my team for helping me to see the Truth through it all; to my daughter, Shayla, for reminding me to play; to my Mom and Dad for my first survival tips; to my colleagues and mentors, Dr. Cynthia and the Burmese Refugee Medics, Bob Condon, Dr's John Titus, Lee Lipsenthal, Wendy Kohatsu, Walt Mills, Jim Gude, Lou Menachoff, Rick Flinders, Ritch Addison, Colin Kopes-Kerr, Rachel Friedman, Scott Eberly, Rachel Naomi Remen, and Dean Ornish, for their enthusiasm and encouragement; to Lauren Carpenter and Erika Petryszyn for their editing and graphics; and finally to my patients for their understanding and trust.

Most of all thanks to you for still being willing to follow your heart into the field of medicine. May the wisdom you gain from experience carry you forward in the best of ways.

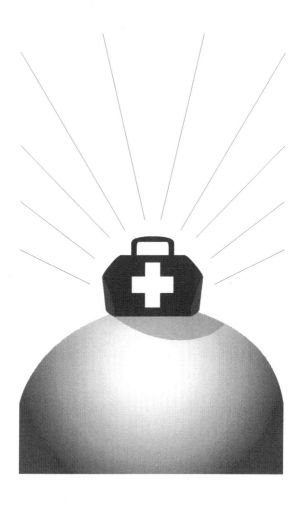

CONTENTS

FOREWORD BY DEAN ORNISH, M.D.

50 Simple Things to Save Your Life During Residency is a game changer for doctors. What I've found in my career is that if you want to make healthy changes, keep it simple. And part of the genius of Ben's book is that it is full of simple tips and wisdom to help you thrive, no matter what life or residency demands of you.

In my experience, there are two types of people who can make something simple: those who know very little about it and make it simplistic, and those who have mastered it and can describe the essence out of a deep understanding, focusing on what's most important. Dr. Ben Brown is clearly in the latter category.

I love this book. Think of it as a survival manual, like a "Worst-Case Scenario" guide for residency. If I had this book during my internship and medical residency at the Massachusetts General Hospital, my life would have been much saner then.

Our understanding of health is changing dramatically. On the one hand, advances in medicine and science have armed physicians with better high-tech treatment options, such as organ transplants and stem cell therapy. On the other hand, our research has proven that making simple changes to your lifestyle can actually reverse heart disease and many other chronic illnesses—an idea considered "impossible" not long ago. In our research, we've used high-tech, expensive, state-of-the-art scientific measurement to prove the power of these simple, low-tech and low-cost interventions.

My colleagues and I also found that these lifestyle changes may stop or even reverse the progression of early-stage prostate cancer. We found that with just three months of a healthier lifestyle more than 500 genes were changed—genes that protect us turned on and genes that promote heart disease, type 2 diabetes, breast cancer, prostate cancer and colon cancer, among others, turned off. Our latest research showed that even our telomeres (the ends of our chromosomes that control aging) get longer and as our telomeres get longer, our lives get longer. Thus, our genes are a predisposition, but our genes are not our fate.

Based on this research, Medicare and major insurance companies are now covering our lifestyle program, helping to create a new financially sustainable paradigm of health care rather than only sick care.

This is all great news. With support to make better choices, people are able to live longer, happier and healthier lives. As doctors, it is incredibly rewarding for us to help our patients prevent and recover from disease. That's why most of us got into this work... we wanted to help people feel better.

If helping others is the reason we got into medicine, the paradox is that our health care training can lead us into a pattern of neglecting our most important resource: our own well-being. Medicine is amongst the noblest of professions and also one of the toughest. Few other vocations demand as much training, expertise, compassion and ability to act under pressure. If we do not find better ways to keep ourselves and our dreams alive, we may forget why we became doctors in the first place.

Residency is where we lay down the foundation for our careers. There's a lot of attention given to mastering the "practice" of medicine, such as reading EKGs, balancing acid-base disturbances or learning a new procedure, but very little guidance on how to live a healthy, joyful life while practicing medicine. I recall my own medical training and the feelings of isolation and burnout it created and how I hungered for something different for myself and my patients.

I've always been troubled by this paradox. If we are to create a health revolution, shouldn't we begin with ourselves? Studies show that you are five to ten times more likely to help your patients make healthy changes if you are living them yourself. We need to embody the core values that we teach others. The best teacher is a good example.

I first met Ben nearly 20 years ago, when he was still in residency. He impressed me with his ability to remain cheerful and optimistic no matter what came his way. _50 Simple Things to Save Your Life During Residency_ shows how he did it in an engaging, humorous and easy-to-digest way. It covers all the key areas of wellness as they apply to the unique challenges of medical residency: nutrition, rest, activity, joy, learning and love.

There has never been a more important time for you to keep your dreams alive in the field of medicine. You have in your hands an outstanding guide to survive residency and beyond. Oh, the places you'll go!

Dean Ornish, M.D.
Founder and President,
Preventive Medicine Research Institute

Clinical Professor of Medicine,
University of California, San Francisco
Author of _The Spectrum_ (and others)

www.ornish.com

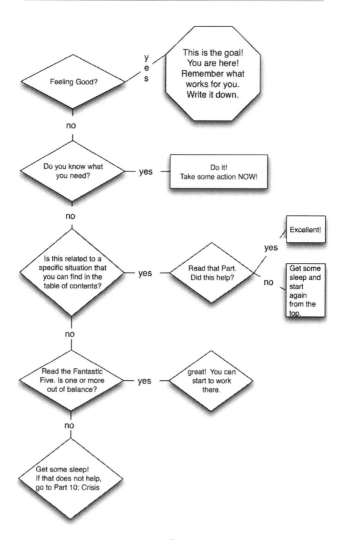

INTRODUCTION

Congratulations, you've just graduated from medical school and are ready to take on the world.

As you wrap your stethoscope around your neck and put that pager on your waist, your world shifts. People begin to call you "Doctor So-and-So" (and it takes a moment to realize that they are referring to you). Nurses follow the orders that you write down (and if you're nice they might tell you what you really wanted to order).

As you walk down the wards you feel a thrill going through your veins; it is so real, so palpable. Then you realize that thrill is your pager set on vibrate. It's the Emergency Room calling, it's time to go do your first admission.

When you hit the ER, you feel like you're in a movie. It is happening so fast that you desperately want a copy of the script. Before you start to panic, realize that you are a star or you wouldn't be here. And if you already knew how to do everything, you also wouldn't be here.

Welcome to Residency, a multi-year long thriller mixed with horror, drama, adventure and romance (if you're lucky). It will likely be one of the most challenging times of your life. You'll work long hours and meet interesting people. You are the star (sorry, no dress rehearsal). If you start to get a bit of stage fright you can take a deep breath, force a smile and realize one of your first tools ... denial. "Hey, this movie's not too bad. I'm a great doctor."

INTRODUCTION

This book is a simple guide to help you navigate through Residency with grace and aplomb. It was written by someone who has been through it himself (yeah, I also walked to the hospital each day uphill both ways and all), but more importantly I have learned from the hundreds of residents just like you who made the most of their experience ... and stayed alive! As Director of Integrative Medicine, Global Medicine and Career Development at one of the University of California San Francisco's Residency programs I get to live the 50 Simple Things every day.

How to Use This Book

You can read this book front to back, back to front, jump right to the section that is most troublesome for you, open to a random page, follow the Residency treatment flow diagram or work through the Fantastic Five pillars of a great Residency.

50 Simple Things gives you easy but powerful tips to preserve your body and make the most of your time in and out of the hospital. It was

designed for you to keep in your pocket so that you can refer to it in moments of downtime and need.

This book is a part of a larger program designed to mentor medical residents and people interested in simple wellness, practicing medicine with integrity and keeping their dreams alive. Please join us at www.theintegrativementor.com. Now, welcome to your first patient ... ahem, that's you.

"You will do foolish things, but do them with enthusiasm!" -Colette

THE
FANTASTIC
FIVE

There are five pillars that will, if done moderately well, keep you and your dreams alive. If you do nothing else, find the best ways for you to get good rest/sleep, move your body, fuel your body, connect with supportive people and cultivate a sense of purpose.

The following index gives you easy access to simple things related to each of the Fantastic Five.

The Fantastic Five

1. **Good Sleep and Relaxation:** get enough sleep and find a simple, healthy way to relax daily. (1,2,5,6,9,13,14,16,20,26,27,29,36,40,41)

2. **Movement and Play:** discover some movement you like to do, build it into your life, and do it often. (7,18,19)

3. **Fuel:** stay well fed, oxygenated and hydrated. (8,15,35)

4. **Loving Supportive Connections:** WARNING: you can't do this alone! Have at least one person who you can confide in, even if you have to hire them ... I mean like a therapist! (Appendix iii, 4,33)

5. **Purpose, Meaning, and Depth:** make sense of this phase of your life and training. (11,17,23,24,25,32,42,45,46,47,48)

PART 1:
POST-CALL

We are starting with simple things you can do post-call, because this is the time when you will be most exhausted physically and emotionally.

It would be simple to just say CHOOSE SLEEP, but there are times when life demands something else. Then a few other simple things are needed. When needed, do them, then choose sleep. May you find the right thing until your head hits the pillow ... and remember tomorrow is a fresh day.

1. Choose Sleep

Take the time post-call to thank your body for all you put it through, ask for its forgiveness, and give it the reward of sleep.

Most people need somewhere around six to eight hours a day. Research shows that seven is a good number to shoot for, but this is highly variable. One of the residents I worked with needed 12 hours to feel good and another only needed five.

You can get tremendous benefits from brief naps (like feeling human again). Though a full sleep cycle takes about 90 minutes, even five minutes of horizontal time can give you a boost. If you like data, studies show that a 20 minute nap is ideal. Personal experience from many say it's best to finish napping by 5:00 p.m. if you want a to go to sleep at a normal time.

There are times of day that are more natural to gently fall asleep. In the evening it is 10:00 p.m. and the daytime it is 11:00 a.m.

Some do very well with a pre-sleep routine: this might include a warm shower, rubbing oil on your feet (a great relaxer), meditation, a pillow screaming session or a glass of warm milk.

If you have trouble getting enough sleep, learn to wind down earlier and ride your first tired wave into bed.

I remember walking into the call room and finding one of my co-residents spread out on the floor fast asleep; it looked like he had been shot mid-step. He rode the first wave out and though he did not make it to the bed, he did wake up refreshed. Ahhh!

2. Nurture Yourself

Take a bath by candlelight, hang out with understanding folks you love, hang out alone, get a massage—set aside time to listen inside and to do what it is that you need to do.

If you don't know how to nurture yourself, ask a few others how they do it.

Notes on How I Nurture Myself

3. Know When You Are Too Tired to Drive

Friends don't let friends drive post-call (when they have not slept).

If you are wondering if you are too tired to drive, here are a few clues:

- **You are starting to hallucinate.** If you see small animals or other objects that aren't really there jumping from the side of the road, time to pull over and sleep.

- **You catch yourself after a head bob.** Be grateful that you did not crash and get off the road.

- **You actually fall asleep waiting for a red light to turn green.** Get off the road!!!!

4. No Charged Conversations Post Call!!!

Post call is a great time for many things (sleep, a haircut, massage, toothbrushing, hot tub, sauna), but it is not a great time to have a confrontational conversation with your co-worker or a button-pushing duel with your significant other.

Note: it is somewhat likely that you will be reading this after violating Simple Thing #4. It's happened to the best of us. Like so many things … just do your best to remember this for next time and do what many others have done, show your 'sparring partner' this page.

5. Release Your Emotions

You will be surrounded by more intense, powerful, life-changing experiences in 24 hours than most people experience in a decade. On the one hand, this is why we are here. On the other hand, this is why some people in medicine go numb. If you do not want to go numb, learn to release your emotions.

Emotions are 'E'-motions, where E stands for energy. That energy needs motion or it can potentially eat someone up. Be creative; find what the energy you're feeling needs and then give it a movement that helps it flow.

Journal, swear, exercise, release, dance, scream, run, sweat, jump, play, stomp, cry, laugh, talk to your friends: most of the time I prefer these activities to drinking, smoking, cussing or punching a wall. Find what works for you, and do it.

6. Get Three Hours of "Instant Sleep"

If you need to perform and are feeling exhausted, here are a few tricks to help recharge without sleep.

- **Brush your teeth** (worth about 30 minutes).

- **Take a shower** (worth about an hour).

- **Jog in place** for one to five minutes (worth about 30 minutes) or go for a run, walk, or bike ride outside (worth about an hour).

- **Do the deep relaxation nap** see #27 Power Nap (worth about an hour).

TOTAL: 3+ hours

Note: the effect is temporary. This is to help you get your 'must do's' done and make it safely to bed.

OK, I know it's not the same as a good snooze, but work with me here. Try it!

PART 2:
GETTING OFF
TO A GOOD START

You will have no idea what each day will bring. Chances are pretty good that many things will be out of your control: what food is available, how late you have to work, how fast you have to move. A few simple practices in the morning can assure you of at least one good meal, some healthy movement and a thicker emotional buffer.

7. Choose Some Movement You Love and Do It Right When You Get Up

Keep it simple, make it fun, build it into your routine and do it often...

Just a few minutes of vigorous or gentle flowing movement can help you "get up on the right side of the bed" and prepare your body and mind for anything.

Be creative here and do what you love! If you love to dance, put on some of your favorite music and go for it. If you like to cycle, bike to work or get an exercise bike/bike trainer.

You may want to get a stationary bike, treadmill, or rebounder in the call room. You can also make friends with the folks in the Physical Therapy Department.

Movement Tips:

- **Make your movement choices as portable as possible.** Get a bike that you can put in or on your car, have your running

21

shoes with you, carry your in-line skates, surf board, etc.

- **Timing:** Most people have found before work, mid day, or before you go home to be the best time to walk, ride your bike or skate. Even better if you can commute this way.

- **Combine movement with connecting with friends or people you want to meet.**

- **Combine other stationary activities with exercise:** Reading, listening to music or a podcast, watching a movie, opening mail, watching a TV show, or CME DVD. I have a friend who rigged up his exercise bike to hold his laptop so he can email while he cycles.

- **Be creative!** Do walking meetings, do exercise on call, have fun...

P.S. Consult with your doctor-self before engaging in any exercise program.

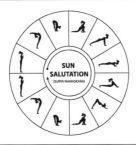

Time Crunch? Three Minute Stretch

Start Standing: Do a Sun Salutation.

Then go onto your back: With your knees bent, let your knees fall to one side and feel the twist, then do the other side. Then pull your knees to your chest and roll around like a ball.

Then sit up: Let your neck relax forward and slowly-gently do a half circle with your head, stop at the top and change direction.

Now you have done a full body stretch in 3 minutes!

Common Sense Note: this is a stretch, stop or back off from any pain and do not do a stretch that is painful.

Time Crunch? Four Minute Interval

Stay fit in four minutes a day with interval training by biking, running in place, or any movement where you can really push yourself.

- **Start slow** and build up to near maximum effort for about one minute.

- **Relax,** catch your breath, take a 2-4 min break or stretch.

- **Repeat** three more times either right now or at different times during the day.

That is it!

Four minutes of high intensity movement like this can be as good for your heart as 30 minutes of continuous jogging or biking.

If you vary your activity every month or so, this type of interval routine can take you a long way!

On a Budget?

<u>No Equipment Needed</u>: dancing (except maybe a stereo), running in place, walking, stretching...

<u>Minimal Equipment</u>: Exercise DVD/YouTube, Rebounder, Yoga, Thera-band...

My Movement Ideas

8. Supercharged Breakfast: Smoothies!
Make 3 Meals in 10 Minutes

Smoothies are super fast, super easy and a super good way to start the day.

Here is my favorite recipe. I make this on most days, and with practice it takes about five minutes to prepare. If I add protein powder and oils, this will last me until lunch. All portions are approximate.

First put seeds, liquid and fruit in a blender...

- 1-2 TBS flax or chia seeds

- ½ cup sunflower seeds (or other nuts)

- 12-16 ounces water (+/- juice=sweeter)

- ½ cup of fruit (e.g. half a banana and a few frozen berries)

Start to blend on low and then turn to high until smooth (I do this first to grind the flax seeds and fruit before adding the powders and oil).

Then add powders, greens and oils

- 2 huge scoops whey protein (or other protein, e.g. rice, hemp, etc.)

- 1 handful leafy greens (like kale, chard, lettuce, etc.) or 1 scoop green powder (I like Pure Synergy or Vitamineral Green)

- If you get hungry before noon add a little oil - I like Udo's Oil, about 2 TBS

Blend until mixed and smooth, yum! You can double or triple the recipe, drink some now and store the rest for later.

Super Charged Smoothie Table

USE ONE OR MORE of each: liquid, protein, healthy oil, +/- sweet, misc., flavor, and then mix.

A little more smoothie Magic...

To boost flavor add a little of either lemon juice, ginger (root or powder), chocolate powder or cardamom...Experiment.

Ingredients	Option 1	Option 2	Option 3
Liquid	Water	Juice & Water	Milk: Rice, Soy or Almond. Kefir
Protein	Nuts or Seeds	Powders	Both
Healthy Oil	Udo's Oil	Add Flax or Chia Seeds	Walnut
If You Need It A Little Sweeter	Dates	Berries: Fresh or Frozen	Banana
Misc	Spinach, Kale or Other Greens	Green Powders	Probiotics
Flavor	Cardamom	Ginger	Lemon

9. Shower Power Meditation

Meditation is much easier than most people realize. It involves four things:

- **Breath:** slow ... rhythmic ... deep.

- **Relaxation:** let go of any worries ... tension ... concerns.

- **Posture:** spine straight ... neck over shoulders.

- **Focus:** on a word, on your breath, on a sensation, on the area between your eyebrows, on a beautiful place in nature, etc. (your choice).

You can do this anywhere but the shower is perfect for a short, power meditation!

Shower Power:

Stand with your back straight. Close your eyes half way and focus between your eyebrows. Take a deep breath and exhale with a sigh. Think of everything you are grateful for. Repeat an affirmation or mantra that resonates with you, such as this one: "*Every day and every way I am getting stronger and healthier.*" With some practice you can do this while you wash your hair and body without losing focus. (And if your housemates hear you, just show them this page and smile).

10. Ultra Rapid Daily Planning

Take five minutes in the morning to:

- Look over what you have planned for the day.
- Write down and prioritize to-do's.
- Gather what you need.

Planning ahead can save you 30 minutes or more through the day. (See Time Management in Part 10 for more on this).

My Rapid Planning Steps

---

11. Set an Intention For the Day

"Intentions" help us find deeper purpose in those otherwise routine (and potentially dull) tasks. For example, the clinic shift you have to do becomes an opportunity to practice being in the moment. The co-worker who rubs you the wrong way becomes an opportunity to work with seeing good in everyone. That extra patient they put on your schedule gives you the opportunity to practice unconditional love with appropriate limits...

Or... You can create an intention from any area or anything that you want to focus on:

Special learning areas: physical exam skills, presentation skills, differential diagnosis, efficiency, using more handouts, etc.

Working with your emotions: returning to center, focus on gratitude, moving anger or sadness.

Working on something fun: find a way to practice guitar, get 10,000 steps of movement, etc.

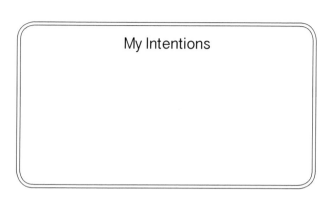

Bonus: Not so simple but powerful… set aside time (five minutes to an hour) for yourself first thing in the morning and combine any of the above into a daily ritual. Do it daily for 30 days and watch your life transform!

My Daily Ritual

PART 3:
IN THE CLINIC

Most residents spend a good chunk of time in the Clinic. For many people, a few "simple things" can make this experience enjoyable or at least less painful. Establishing good patterns here can set you up for a lifetime of good habits, such as learning something new with each patient, honing your skills with agenda setting, practicing how to overcome co-dependent tendencies ... your patients will teach you while you help them.

Clinic is a place where you deepen relationships over time with people that you would otherwise unlikely come in contact with. They will share their lives, joys and struggles with you. Although sometimes the work load and the inefficiencies can make it hard to get through the day, the opportunity to see the world through someone else's eyes, even for a moment, is a privilege.

"The art of happiness is to serve all." - Yogi Tea

12. Arrive Early ...

This is not something that I did naturally! Perhaps you already know the benefits of arriving early, but if not, give it a try and see what it is like.

To succeed in Clinic, you will do much better if you can be prepared.

Try arriving early and go through your check-list to set yourself up for a good day.

Example Daily Checklist:

- Check in with medical assistant

- Review patients

- Relax and breathe

- Eat a snack

13. Door Knob/Chart Breath

I had a mentor who used to say, "*Your peace has to be big enough to hold their pain. Your love has to be bigger than their fear. Your presence has to be able to dance with whatever comes into the room. At least some of the time.*"

When you take the door knob or chart in hand and are about to go into a patient's room:

- Take a deep breath

- Let go of the last patient

- Center yourself

- Be present for this person

- Think of my mentor's mantra (above)

14. Shake Off Bad Mojo

When it feels like a patient or co-worker just emotionally vomited on you or sucked you dry (an emotional vampire) take a few moments to shake it off. Go into the bathroom. Begin by shaking your legs—shake them and let the wave build up to a full-body shake (like a big wet dog). Repeat until you can feel yourself again.

You can also do a ritual cold water shower: wash your hands with cold water and then pretend to be washing your body off with a hand-held shower and make the "shhhh" sound of water. Yeah, I know it sounds kinda Third Grade corny, but just try it. You'll feel better.

15. Snack Break: Tea Time

Even a quick five minute bite can boost your energy until the end of Clinic. Most people will start to konk out at either 11:00 a.m. or 3:00 p.m. Bring and eat healthy snacks, and carry a water bottle or thermos. Sit next to a window, or go outside (if you can) and take some deep breaths. On long days even a one minute break can bring a fresh perspective!

Super Snacks

- Apple with almond butter

- Avocado with soy sauce

- Walnuts, pecans or almonds

- Power Bar of choice

- A little bit of dark chocolate

My List of Snacks

16. Re-frame Your Reality

This is potentially the most powerful tool in this book. How you see it determines how you feel about it!

Re-framing allows you to change how you look at an event and therefore change how you feel. Use this for yourself and your patients.

To the mom whose child was born with an extra finger, it might be very healing for her to know that some cultures view that as a sign of abundance.

To yourself after a rough call night, it might help to think:

"What I learned last night is preparing me for saving someone's life when I am out in practice and do not have the support around."

"Utter and complete exhaustion is the state by which I will reach Nirvana."

"The Chinese symbol for crisis is the same as for opportunity."

You get the idea, be creative and watch how re-framing your perspective changes how you feel.

17. Choose One Project and Take It All the Way Through

Clinic is one place where not everything is as smooth as we would like it, especially if you are working with an underserved population. Find the one thing in Clinic that you really want to see change and give it your best. Do not let it consume you, but work as an individual or a group to help bring change in where it is needed.

My List of Possible Clinic Improvements

PART 4:
IN THE HOSPITAL

The hospital can be wildly satisfying or just wild. People who get admitted to the hospital or come into the emergency room typically have more serious and urgent matters. The work is hard, but on the other hand you get labs back quickly (if you're lucky), you are often working closely with other physicians and you typically have a little more time to think about what someone has going on (that is, after you have mastered where the bathrooms are, where to get your food, how to log onto the computer and where to sleep). The following tips are designed to help you stay present through the barrage of the hospital ...

18. Wear Good Socks and Great Shoes

Do I need to say more? ...Please! As for socks, Thorlos or Smart Wool are great and last forever. If you need more support, get heel pads or arch supports at the local sporting goods store or pharmacy. This will keep a nice spring in your step!

19. Stretch On Rounds

Find a way to do this that respects the team and the patients. It is a great way to keep your body going!

20. Manage Stress Like a Samurai

Face what is stressing you, it is never as scary as it is when we imagine it.

- **Be In the Moment:** You do not have to take it quite to the extreme of the Samurai Warrior who said "*today is a good day to die.*" He meant "*be complete with those you love.*" Leave nothing hanging out there to drain you.

41

- **Re-learn to Breathe:** The Samurai had simple breathing practices to help manage difficult situations. They are very easy to learn and apply.

  - **The Sigh:** The Samurai would use this after a battle. Inhale deeply and let it out with sound.

  - **Counting While Breathing:** The Samurai would use breath counting during sparring sessions to stay relaxed and fluid. You can use it when walking the hospital hallways. Simply count your steps while you inhale and count your steps while you exhale.

  - **Curled Tongue:** When anger struck, a Samurai would breathe through a curled tongue. Try it, it cools you down.

  - **Nostril Alternation:** When fearful, the Samurai would exhale then inhale through the left nostril and then alternate to the right with the next breath.

- **Learning to Let Go:** Some muscles when tense need help to relax, and tensing them first often helps. Tense a muscle and hold to the count of four, then take a deep inhale and relax it with your exhale. The Samurai would use this when a part of the body was not as fluid as it needed to be. For most in the hospital this is our neck and shoulders. Inhale, bring your shoulders up towards your ears, tighten, hold, then exhale and let them go. Ahhhh!

PART 5:
THE ENDLESS DAY: LATE NIGHTS OR ON-CALL

On-call is the most commonly feared part of Residency. Perhaps it is because we fear that we will be revealed to be an "impostor doctor." (Ok, in case you did not know it, most people in medicine have felt, at times, like they are doctor impersonators ... so you are not alone if you feel this way.) The truth is you need to pull together a lot when you are on call and for most people this is nearly impossible early in Residency.

The following tips will help bolster or restore you as "the person" while you are learning to be "the doctor."

In addition to getting good with your differential diagnosis and patient presentations, restore your sanity in between the frames with a few of the simple things in this section.

21. Don't Worry About a "Call Night" Ahead of Time

Who knows what will happen? Perhaps a nuclear bomb or an earthquake will happen and your call night will be canceled. The only way to be disappointed is to have expectations. Let go of your expectations and mentally prepare for the worst case scenario. Then ask the universe for what it is you really want (and trust that you will always get what you need).

22. Don't Make Plans for Post-Call That You Can't Easily Break

It's a good time for dental appointments, haircuts and sleep. It's not a great time for activities that require mental juice.

23. Enjoy Yourself at the Hospital

Since you're there so much, you may as well enjoy yourself. If your day is slow, put your feet up and take a catnap, stretch, exercise, sleep, read or dance. Remember to drink water.

Give each other mini-breaks. Hold the beeper for your co-resident so they can go for a quick run, roller blade in the back parking lot, have dinner with their kids, etc.

Bring in treats for the team.

24. Create a Residency Signature Ritual

We had midnight dance jam. It was started by a class ahead of me and we would all meet in the library at midnight, put on some great music and dance. What will your signature be for your Residency? You can borrow this or invent your own. Exercise under the stars, wheelchair races at midnight, whatever it is, have fun and release for a few minutes before you have to do the next admit or catch a bit of sleep.

25. Live Now

What is it that you love? What makes you feel like life is worth living? Find a way to bring that part of your life into your work and help others to do this too. Work together, create solutions, give more than you take.

```
              What Do You Love?



```

26. Adopt a Mantra or Two for Your Sanity

A mantra is a saying you repeat out loud or silently to yourself. Over time it sinks in and shows up in your life. My two favorites are:

"I am radiant health!" Especially useful to ward off an impending cold.

"All I need is within me now!" Especially useful for when you are walking into an unfamiliar situation.

Or if preparing for impending criticism or self doubt you can use another of my favorites, "F*%# IT!" And watch those feelings disappear.

Others take a saying from their faith or something like, *"Every day and every way I am getting better, better and better."* Have fun with it and watch how it works when you repeat a mantra long enough with concentration and energy.

27. Learn How to Power Nap

This is a *core skill* for Residency survival. It is worth your patience and effort and will pay huge dividends to learn it well. Start by thinking about this as a deep relaxation nap. Over time it will become sleep.

Location: Some residents have a vehicle that they can easily nap in and others find a place in or near the hospital/clinic where they can rest without disruption.

Timing: There are times of day that are more natural to cruise out on, those are generally 11:00 a.m. to 1:00 p.m. and 10:00 p.m. to 2:00 a.m. It's best to finish napping by 5:00 p.m. if you want to go to sleep at a normal time. If you are tired late in the day and can hold out to go to bed until 7:00 p.m., your cycle will normalize faster.

Power Nap Checklist (in or out of hospital):

- **Step One:** *Program your mind* for possible pages/interruptions, and set an alarm for when you have to get up (in case you fall into deep sleep).

49

To program your mind, say something like, *"If I am paged while I am resting, I will wake up gently, alert and ready for any issue and then go back to sleep easily when this issue is handled."*

- **Step Two:** *Put a paper and pen near your bed* in case you remember a "to-do" item as you are drifting off.

- **Step Three:** *Lie in a comfortable position and begin rhythmic deep breathing.* Count your inhale and exhale. Inhale: one, two, three, four. Exhale: one, two, three, four. Inhale: one, two, three, four ... and so on...

  If you are tense in any part of your body, tense it, hold for four seconds and then relax it.

- **Step Four:** *Use one of your senses to carry you deeper.*

  Vision: imagine you are drifting off into a soft cloud that is absorbing any worries or problems and helping you to relax, unwind and let go.

Touch/Feeling: feel yourself sinking into the mattress.

Sound: hear the gentle waves of your breath and imagine it carrying you into a warm calm ocean.

- **Step Five:** *enjoy, practice and modify* as you need and feel the restorative benefits!

28. Master a Few Things

First, get good at presentations and phone medicine. These skills help other people to help you and you are judged more on these two skills than anything else.

Second, get good at triage. This is a simple thing that requires your attention and gets better with experience. Is this patient big sick or little sick? Is this problem urgent, emergent, or can it wait?

Third, have a few ways to create new thoughts about a Differential Diagnosis, (V-I-N-D-I-C-A-T-E-S, etc.) You can find these in most hospital handbooks.

Lastly, learn one or two conditions really well. You should know them well enough that you can teach your team and perhaps even your Attendings.

One thing most people have trouble with is how to practice good phone medicine, so I will include it here.

Six Keys to Phone Medicine:

When talking to an Attending or Consultants: anticipate interruptions and say less.

1. **Check in:** *"Do you have a minute to ... "*

2. **Tell them what they are listening for.** Why are you calling them and what do you want them to listen for: e.g. a possible admission, antibiotic recommendations, etc.

3. **Ask, "Do you want a brief or complete presentation?"** They will ask for a brief presentation most of the time and they expect a flow of information that roughly follows: age, sex, subjective info, objective info, impression, plan, and questions.

4. **Always finish up your patient presentation with your plan and restate your questions.**

5. **Ask about the longer-term plan.** This is for your learning as well as for your efficiency. For example: *"How long do patients with pancreatitis generally stay in the hospital? When do you start them on liquids? Do you re-check their amylase and lipase?"* etc.

6. **Finish with "Is there anything you want to be called about?"** It makes them think and almost always leads to high yield learning. It also helps you relax if you end up having to call about one of the things they mentioned at 4:00 a.m.

My Late Night/On-Call Things to Do

PART 6:
BETWEEN THE FRAMES

You can wait for those big chunks of time to do the things you love and want to be doing. Sad thing is that they are as elusive as they are longed for and do not materialize as often as we want in Residency.

In order to create a life that works, we have to change our expectations and our approach.

- That one to two hour gym trip can become a 20 minute power workout, so that when you have the one to two hour break you can pull into the gym without pulling a muscle.

- Those long study sessions of medical school become short bursts of study in between scheduled events.

- The wandering in the woods for a few hours can become a really relaxing 10 minute jaunt.

If we let creativity flow, then what we need, want or love is ready for us when that little break arrives.

29. Walking Meditation

In between the frames, we walk. You can add three things to turn your mandatory travel into a meditation and arrive relaxed and ready for whatever life brings: breath, relaxation, and posture...

Three Keys to turn a Walk into a Meditation

- **Breath:** Slow ... rhythmic ... deep.

- **Relaxation:** Let go of any worries ... tension ... concerns.

- **Posture:** Spine straight, neck over shoulders.

That is all there is to it. It is easy and effective! With practice you can vary the speed. You might even try counting steps with your inhale and exhale or repeating a saying that you like to the pace of your steps. Experiment. Make it work for you and have fun doing it!

30. Carry One Book or One Article

When you have downtime or you get somewhere early or the person you are meeting is running late, pull out your reading material and learn, relax, and enjoy.

31. Have a Strategy for Fat Times and Thin Times

An hourglass is a nice metaphor. Life is always going to involve times where you have a relative abundance of free time (fat times) and times where you have a relative deficit of free time (thin times).

It is particularly important to make a plan during fat times for how you are going to keep your life's passions alive in the thin times.

Knowing what your passions are is a great start! Remembering them is much harder when you have precious free moments. Being prepared to do them is even harder.

This is a practice that you can build over time. It will make your life hum, even when it's thin! *Also see Time Management in Part 10 : Appendix

32. Trickle Your Passions

Residency sometimes feels like being force-fed your favorite food. Choosing to balance your life can restore sanity and make you much easier to be around for your non-medical friends.

If you have a passion to serve, that is great. If you have a creative activity you love to do, that is perfect. If you want to learn something new, excellent.

When you know what you love, find a way to do it.

Here are a few suggestions:

- Make what you love as portable as possible.

- Find ways to exercise your passion in one minute, five minutes, or 15 minutes or more.

- Do two things you love at the same time (like exercise and talk to a friend).

- Combine your passion with other activities you don't love to make them more fun when possible (like listening to music and doing a chair dance while finishing charts).

My Ideas to Tickle My Passion

33. As Ye Sow, So Shall Ye Reap

This is the law of cause and effect.

- **Treat every patient with dignity and respect.** The paradox is that in doing this you will feel more human.

- **Be good to the nurses and receptionists.** Lets face it, you've had more school and they've had more experience. Listen and learn from them, and let them help you. Be a team and all will benefit. They will save your butt at least as many times as they wake you up for something that probably could wait.

- **When you smile and are pleasant against all evidence, it comes back to you.** So do your other behaviors ...

- **Make it fun.** Connect with and create opportunities to socialize with your colleagues.

PART 7:
MAKING THE MOST OF YOUR EVENINGS

Evenings are like gold if you have done the things that let you throw the "off switch" to work. If there is any part of your work that you are going to take with you, handle it quickly, let it go and then get away. (No, this is not always possible, but do your best.)

Then go and enjoy a meal with a friend, take a bath, get a massage, give a massage, enjoy your sweet friends and the activities that fill you up again ...

34. Work on What is Needed

Look at your life! Then work on the area that you need to build the most, and have some fun doing it too!

A good start is to review the Fantastic Five in the front of this book ...

- Good Sleep and Relaxation

- Movement

- Fuel

- Connection

- Purpose, Meaning, and Depth

My Common Needs

35. Great Food Fast

Dr. Ben's Simple Blender Soup

- Look in the fridge. What produce do you have that needs to be eaten before it goes bad?

- Toss it in the blender first then add any of the following: carrots, celery, tomatoes, avocado.

- Add some nuts, a bit of olive oil, a cube of bullion, any other spices you like

- Add some hot water and blend!

Dr. Ben's Toaster Oven Taco

- Get a tortilla (flour or corn)

- Open a can of refried or whole beans and smear a bit on the tortilla

- Cut up a few strips of cheese and put those on the beans and pop in the toaster oven, like you would a piece of toast (best if you have a little tray you can put it on).

- When the cheese is melted, enjoy! Add as you like some salsa, avocado/guacamole, sprouts, lettuce, tomatoes, etc.

Super Fast Asian Wrap

This recipe comes courtesy of Solana (thanks!). I like it because it requires very few ingredients, is super fast and is a great way to eat more veggies without stuffing yourself with a salad. You will have to get rice paper at an Asian market.

- Edible Rice paper wrap (Bánh tráng)

- Pre-washed salad mix

- Nuts (any kind)

- Olive oil or some type of tasty dressing

- Leftovers: Tomatoes, cucumbers, avocados, sliced tofu, chicken or anything else you like

- Get all your ingredients ready to put in your wrap (once the rice paper is wet it will get sticky fast).

- Wet your rice paper, put in the ingredients, wrap it up quickly.

- Cut it (if you want) and eat. Yum!

Favorite Food Ideas

36. Go Off the Grid

Want a mini-retreat at home? Turn off the phone and pager and take a mini-vacation (note: may not want to do this if on call). These mini-vacations can be two minutes or an evening. The key is the 3 R's: Relax, Recover and Recharge. This may be best done alone or with others.

If you have a little more time and you are prepared you can get away for the night. Ask your friends, the local sports shop or camping gear place for nearby hot spots.

Pick four or five places less than an hour away to relax, unwind, sleep, stretch, have a nice meal or meditate. Rent a motel-room, camp or sleep in your car (if it's big enough), just get away. The hospital and your patients will survive without you.

List of Get-Away Places within an Hour

37. Simplify Your Life

Spend as little of your free time as possible doing things you don't like. You may want to consider getting a cleaning service, creating less mess, hiring an organizer, etc.

List for Simplifying

- Get rid of ⅓ of your stuff

- Throw away your journals

- Stop junk mail

- Buy a washer and dryer

- Finish two projects

My List of Simplifying

38. Organize Your Learning

- **Very simple.** Study at the time when you are seeing patients. Jot down notes for further study and spend 10 minutes at the end of your day looking these up.

- **Learn a few resources that work well for you.** I love books. I love it when information is presented visually. We all learn in different ways, find your way and find reference material that spoon-feeds you in your way.

- **The Basics: Organizing Files.** Be a minimalist on files, but keep the important stuff, store items alphabetically, get rid of hanging files, use a labeler, and set aside time to do them all at once (see the book *Getting Things Done* by David Allen for more info). I also recommend creating an electronic filing cabinet and using it the same way. Scan everything you can and carry it on a flash drive or your phone.

- **Less Simple: Peripheral Brain**. If you have not heard of a peripheral brain then this can be revolutionary. It is basically a customized "notebook" of things that you want to remember. Door codes, phone numbers, and passwords are obvious contents, but you can also put in how to do a discharge summary, how to treat headaches or any other thing that is difficult to recall and important to recall when you need it.

  - **Digital Linear People.** Make notes in a computer or smartphone.

  - **Visual Tactile People.** Take notes in an appropriately sized notebook. (Moleskine makes several sturdy options.) I recommend organizing it alphabetically. The benefit of referring back to the same thing frequently is that it helps the learning sink in fast and deep.

PART 8:
WEEKEND REJUVENATORS AND VACATIONS

For anyone seeking excellence, recharging your batteries when you have more time is essential. Staying alive, or more specifically keeping your passions alive, during Residency means turning work off and returning to what you love or what you need right now. This might be the time to fit in a two hour workout or walk in the woods. It might also be the time to sleep in or take a nap. Enjoy and be a little selfish here, it will pay dividends to all those who know you.

39. Get Out of Town!

Make a List of Places to get away to that are (preferably) less than four hours away.

Then ask the question, "What do I need most right now?" Don't get too conceptual with your answers. Instead, focus on specific things you can do that are healing, for example: sleep, a hike in nature, healthy meals with lots of vegetables.

My Special Get-Aways (Semi-Secret)

40. Have a Physical and Emotional Outlet

Physical and emotional energy can be creative, sustaining or destructive. If you do not give your energy an outlet, it will become destructive. You need to find ways to keep your energy moving so that it can work for you rather than against you. The easiest ways to move your energy are to move your body and engage in activities that you love to do. It's really that easy!

Suggestions if Your Main Emotion is:

- **Anger:** Release it with vigorous exercise. Anger stimulates the muscles in our arms so give them a workout—throw modeling clay (or your pager) at the wall, punch the air, do push-ups, etc. Stimulate your sense of humor by learning a new joke a day or playing games.

- **Sadness:** Get up and get active—take a walk, get together with good friends, work on what you have been putting off, start a hobby or renew an old one, pray for your friends. Drink a mug of green tea chai.

73

- **Fear:** Relax your nervous system: bathe by candlelight, rub oil on your body (sesame oil—raw not roasted—or coconut oil), stay warm, eat regular meals, avoid coffee, and get sleep.

Also ... your right brain is the seat of creativity and emotional expression. Try painting, clay work, drumming, dancing, reading or writing short stories, poetry, a dream diary, a journal or whatever works for you to express and release what you are feeling.

41. Schedule An SFMD

WTF is an SFMD? It's Spontaneous-Flow-Magic Day (SFMD) or a Self Medicine Day/Conference.

This is a time where you make no plans and use the time as you wish: putter around the house, catch up on sleep, take a bike ride, spend the day in nature, read a book for pleasure, or what ever spontaneous activity makes you hum in the moment.

It's important to schedule at least a half hour SFMD meeting a week and one longer conference each quarter. They will recharge you and give you the mental space necessary so that you can be your best for both your patients and yourself.

How to Take an SFMD:

- **Pick a day or afternoon that is open.** Type/Write SFMD in your calendar.

- **Guard it like gold.** When anyone asks you to do something that day, look at your calendar and say, *"I would love to but I have a conference that day."* This is great if they are looking over your shoulder, it is right there looking at both of you.

42. Annual Retreat

I am a huge proponent of taking a three day solo retreat at least once each year. Use this time off alone to define your vision for the next year. Summer is probably the best time for this, but any time is better then not.

43. Vacation

Plan to take at least two vacations per year. It's important that you take at least seven days off in a row to really unwind. Here is the nearly universal resident experience.

- Day one to three of vacation: lay a bit low and sleep a lot while you ride the emotions that come and go.

- Over the next few days: feel parts of your personality you thought were long gone come back. Watch, Feel, Enjoy!!!!

44. Be Creative With Your Time Off

"On Call for your holiday? Don't despair!" - Have Christmas or Chanukah a day late; celebrate your birthday on your day off, etc. Remember that everyone feels low in December & January; schedule your vacation to the tropics then.

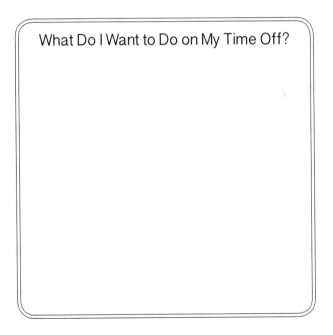

What Do I Want to Do on My Time Off?

PART 9:

THE LIGHT AT THE END OF THE TUNNEL-PREPARING TO GET OFF THE TRACK

If you are in your first year of Residency you may think this section is not for you. Think again! Even if you are in medical school or done with Residency, these simple strategies can allow you to fund your own sabbatical, plan your elective time, find a mentor or simply give a part of you that feels anemic a little transfusion.

"I'm looking forward to looking back on all this."
-Sandra Knell

45. Point Yourself in the Direction of Your Passions

You can have what you really want. Entertain your most amazing life.

46. Re-Read Your Personal Statement

This is a great way to remind yourself why you did this!

47. Know the Difference Between a Job and Your Work. Create a Hybrid Life if Needed

Job: Something that is good enough and pays the bills.

Work: What you were put here to do!

48. Hang Onto Your Dream

The moment you stop dreaming, you stop living. Keep living your dreams no matter what, and wait out the hard parts. You are standing on the shoulders of those who have gone before you, and someone else may stand on yours. If you do not do your part then they will have no shoulders to stand on.

My Most Extravagant Medical Dream

49. Know Thyself

It is said that professional training puts our emotional development about 10 years behind our peers. I am not so sure I agree. I suppose it depends what our peers have been doing during that time. We often see more tragedy in one shift than most will see in a lifetime and yet we typically do not take the time to digest it, seek deeper meaning, and learn from what we go through. This is a plug to do that. Learn from what you have been through and get to know the depth of who you are and then live that! (Need some ideas? Go back to Parts 7 and 8.)

50. Plan For Post-Residency Recovery Time

Start early and set aside money for post-Residency vacation and recovery.

After Residency, most people are ready for a mini-sabbatical. You will know how long you need, but if you are only planning for several weeks, please rethink your plan.

How to save for your first mini-sabbatical: set an amount that gets automatically deposited into an account that you don't touch, then over the course of your Residency you can squirrel away a sizable nut. Calculate your loan payments and monthly cost of living for the amount of time you will want to be free from responsibility. Start saving now.

Here are some examples of post-Residency vacations and sabbaticals to get your juices flowing ...

Post Residency Recovery Examples

- Took a year to do volunteer work in Burma

- Traveled to Australia and SCUBA dove at the Great Barrier Reef

- Hiked the entire Pacific Crest Trail

- Volunteered in Africa and returned to teach others about it

- Had a baby

- Got married and went to South America on a sail boat

- Went to France for a month with the entire graduating class

PART 10:
APPENDIX

- Time Management

- Crisis

- Relationships

- Kids

Appendix i: TIME MANAGEMENT

Time is on your side ... (or it can be). Time is a paradox; your time is both abundant and limited. Manage it like a philanthropist manages money. You have 24 hours a day. Where do you need to be and where do you want to gift your time?

Time Management Principles

- **One Place:** Keep all calendar items and to-do's (work and personal) in one place and customize it to fit your needs.

- **Two Options:** People generally lean towards either a digital-linear or visual-tactile notational style. If you do not have a system you already like, I recommend a planner pad for visual-tactile people and a smartphone for digital-linear folks.

- **Three Actions:**
  Daily: 5 minutes in the morning:
  Look at your calendar and to do lists.
  Gather supplies needed.

Weekly: 20 minutes on Friday or Sunday. Look ahead two weeks and plan for your week.
Monthly: Review your list of Passions, Goals, or Resolutions if you have one.

The Four Levels of Time Management Needs.

Consider Growing or shrinking your system as your needs change. If what you are doing is working, great. If not, then it is time to go up a level.

- **Level 1: No System:** Remember the important stuff in your head.

- **Level 2: Calendar and List Management:** Put all your activities and to-do's in one place.

  Put any fixed activity in the calendar and then review each morning and prepare for those activities.

  Write down your to-do's on daily and/or weekly lists and prioritize them.

Assign items an A, B, or C based on what is most important to move you towards success. Do your A's before your B's

- **Level 3: Project Management:** Organize more complex groups of activities and ongoing changing priorities/lists. Review and adjust on a daily, weekly, monthly, quarterly basis until done.

- **Level 4: Life Management:** Look at your life categories/roles/goals and develop an ongoing strategy to make major movement in that direction. In general, I recommend getting some coaching or training to move to this level.

Appendix ii. CRISIS

- Acute Personal Crisis Moments

"In the middle of difficulty lies opportunity."
-Albert Einstein

- **Find humor in a crisis and learn to laugh at yourself.** If you are going to laugh about it in 10 years, laugh about it now.

- **Affect (mood) is contagious.** Surround yourself with people you want to be like or get out into nature.

- **Release.** Go into a bathroom and shadow box, cry or scream into a pillow.

- **Ask another resident or friend for help.**

- **Meditate, pray or ask the Universe for help.** If you have never meditated or prayed before, Residency is a great time to start. Try reading the *Three-Minute Meditator* by David Harp. As for prayer it helps to believe in a higher power or greater meaning to all of this craziness, but that is not essential. If you have a belief in anything bigger than little old you, just go deeper into that. If not, then try visualization, hypnosis or read Larry Dossey, *The Power of Prayer*. Here's a sample prayer for the weary resident.

Oh higher power grant me the strength to make it through this period of indentured servitude. Please keep the patients healthy enough for the nurses not to call and the ER doc to feel comfortable sending the patient home. Keep my body healthy and my spirit young. Protect me so I can better be there to serve. And keep my life fun. Oh yeah, and if we could get some Thai food before the night's up that would be great. Thanks!

- Chronic Crisis

"In an abnormal situation, abnormal behavior is normal behavior." -Victor Frankel

"Sometimes we turn to God when our foundations are shaking only to find it is God who is shaking them." -Anonymous

If you wanted to make an intelligent, creative person depressed, you might design a life for them where they:

- Had to stay up really late and go through emotionally challenging experiences with no time to process.

- Keep them from most of their friends and family.

- Keep them so busy that they could not find time for their hobbies.

- Feed them hospital food.

- Make them spend most of their time with sick people.

Sound familiar?

It is normal to feel overwhelmed and it is normal to feel self-doubt. One exercise to stop over-generalizing your self-doubt is the three column rational response.

- **First Column:** List your thought (e.g.. *"I gave the wrong medicine, therefore I'm a bad person, and therefore I will never be a good doctor."*)

- **Second Column:** List your thought pattern (e.g. magnification, over generalization, etc.).

- **Third Column:** List a rational conclusion thought (e.g. *"I gave the wrong medicine, therefore I need to read up on CHF or talk more to my attendings."*)

If you have a lot of self-deprecating thoughts you may want to read *Feeling Good* by David Burns.

- **Learn to say NO.** Set limits on how much is too much. The best way to say No is to be honest with your reality. An example to your superior might be, *"If you would like me to do that, then which one of the things that I am currently responsible for would you like me to drop?"*

- **A perfectionist's path leads to an early grave and there are many disappointing bumps along the way...** You can no longer learn it all, and you will make mistakes. To expect perfection is a set up for failure. I recommend shooting for excellence instead. The perfectionist mantra from Rachel Remen, *"Anything worth doing is worth doing half-assed!"*.

- **Pick one major focus outside of work and commit to it.** It could be Tai Chi, yoga, a relationship, etc. Just pick one and commit to it.

- **Find a role model or select elements of folks you admire as your role model.** You may even want to ask someone to be your mentor for a project or activity. They will likely be flattered and may even be willing to do it.

- **Have a vision.** Go back to your original reasons for becoming a doctor (perhaps re-reading your personal statement will trigger those neurons). This is a great time to be an idealist. My reasons go something like, "*I want to be the kind of doctor I would want my family go to, to be the type of resident I would want to work with, and to help create a world worth living in.*" Choose activities that support your vision.

- **Build a support system and go to a support group** (or start a support group if one doesn't exist). There is a time for planting, a time for cultivating, and a time for harvesting.

- **Planting:** choose to spend your time with those you respect and who respect you.

- **Cultivating:** Spend time with friends when you don't need them. Be there for each other.

- **Harvesting:** Call on friends when you do need them.

This is a natural cycle, do your best. It helps to keep the people in your life feeling valued and not used. You'll find that co-dependency shifts to interdependence.

Special Notes:

The darkest time of Internship is December to February. It will likely never be as dark again.

If these tips are not helping, seek professional help!

Appendix iii. RELATIONSHIPS

- **Get your lives in sync as much as possible and get away together.** If your partner is in Residency or also very busy, try to schedule things so that your up times and your off times are occasionally the same.

- **Make love in the middle of the day** so that neither of you are too tired.

- **Teach your partner what it is you do.**

- **You both have to be brave and learn to ask for what you need.** No mind-reading expectations!

- **Block out time to spend together each week.**

- **Post call is the most critical time.** No—I repeat—no emotionally charged talks post-call. Table it until you have slept. And no dishes either. You are fit to be spoiled and little else.

- **Acknowledge and be grateful for the things you do for each other.**

- **Answer spouse's/SO's pages promptly.** Develop a code system. (E.g. 777 = just thinking about you, your tel# = call when you can, and tel# with a 1 or 911 at the end of it = call ASAP).

- **Don't get divorced until at least 6 months after Residency.** If you can stand waiting you might find a major shift when you've had a chance to be yourself again.

- **If you must marry during Residency** do so, but marry a supremely understanding, empathetic and independent mate.

- **Suggested reading:**
  Getting the Love You Want, Harville Hendricks; *Conscious Loving*, Gay and Kathlyn Hendricks; *Hold Me Tight*, Sue Johnson

Our Ideas to Make it Work and Keep it Fun!

Appendix iv: KIDS

"We Tibetans love all ceremonial and elegant dress; and, perhaps even more important, as a national characteristic we love a joke...We are what Westerners call easy-going and happy-go-lucky by nature, and it is only in the most desperate circumstances that our sense of humor fails us." -His Holiness the Dalai Lama of Tibet

- **Pay attention to what's going on inside of them.** Children are all unique and have different needs. Get to know what they like and want.

- **Show them that you love them even when you can't spend as much time with them as you would like.** Call or FaceTime, bring them to the hospital, have dinner with them when you are on call. Get the support of others to bring them by when you are at work; they will remember it for the rest of their lives.

- **Be there for the important things.** Pick three or four events that you won't miss and do what you have to do to be there.

- **Be compassionate with them and they will be compassionate with you.** Also be compassionate with yourself.

- **Scrap cleaning for the next few years.** It is much more important to be with them than to have a clean house. And they may like the dirt.

- **Talk to others with kids.** Learn what to do and what not to do.

- **Get a babysitter who you can rely on.** Then plan some time away with each of your kids one-on-one at least twice a year.

- **Keep life simple.** This is your main focus outside of work. Let them know it and do not add a lot of other stuff until after Residency. Also don't fill their lives so that you and your partner are running around trying to get them here and there when you are off.

- **Get into their world.** Sit with them, read to them, listen to them, play games. Think about what they are doing even when you are at the hospital, send emails, make calls, send love even when you can't call.

- **Let them teach you how to play again!** Check out the book *Playful Parenting* by Lawrence Cohen.

My Ideas to Love My Kid(s)

Epilogue:

It all starts with individuals staying alive through a challenge. Your passion for medicine will fluctuate and Residency will often feel like you are being force fed your favorite food. It is my hope that this book will help keep you (and subsequently that passion) alive.

So, go forward, watch your behind, and wait out the hard parts. The light at the end of the tunnel will get brighter after every call night.

To your survival,

-Dr. Ben

About the Author:

Ben Brown, M.D. grew up on a farm in Northern California. He graduated from the University of California San Francisco Medical School and from Santa Rosa Community Hospital Family Medicine Residency.

His career in medicine has been a thrilling adventure: from international work (with more than 20 trips around the world and starting two non-profits), to teaching others how to reverse heart disease with Dean Ornish .MD., to mentoring residents as director of Integrative Medicine, Global Medicine, and Career Development at the University of California San Francisco's Santa Rosa Family Practice Residency.

Ben is an award-winning writer, teacher and humanitarian. He enjoys studying the dynamic dance of life, transition, and transformation. In his work and life he strives to remember the spirit by remembering to have fun and love all.

When he is not teaching, seeing patients, or hanging out with his family and friends, you might find him retreating on a nearby mountain, playing his guitar or harmonica, writing in his journal, practicing yoga, juggling glowing balls, biking, roller blading or backpacking.

Save a Life with a Simple Gift

Would you like to give 50 Simple Things to a group of residents who are near and dear to your heart?

We'll make it easy and affordable for you to order copies for all the residents you know. This book makes a great gift for an entire residency class either at the beginning of the year or in the dark of winter.

Simply go to www.theintegrativementor.com and look for the Multiple Copies Button. Feel free to pass this tip along to the chiefs, residency director, or anyone else who would benefit from a class of healthier, happier residents.

This Book Is Part of a Larger Health Care Providers Wellness Project

See what we are up to at ResidentRevolution.com

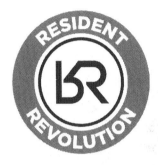

And

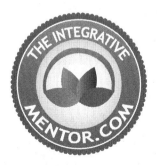

More Pearls of Wisdom?

Do you have a Self-Care Pearl to Share with others?

-Send Us Your Pearls to Share!

Do you have a Question for Us to Answer?

-Please Ask Us Your Questions!

Do you want to see our App Recommendations, Product Reviews and More?

-Sign up for our Newsletter!

We often have free bonuses, so don't be shy!

Ben@theintegrativementor.com

<u>My Simple Notes:</u>

37435149R00066

Made in the USA
San Bernardino, CA
30 May 2019